THE COOKBOOK OF THE

PLANT-BASED PROJECT

Join the Growing Number of People That Are Choosing To Live the Sustainable Way

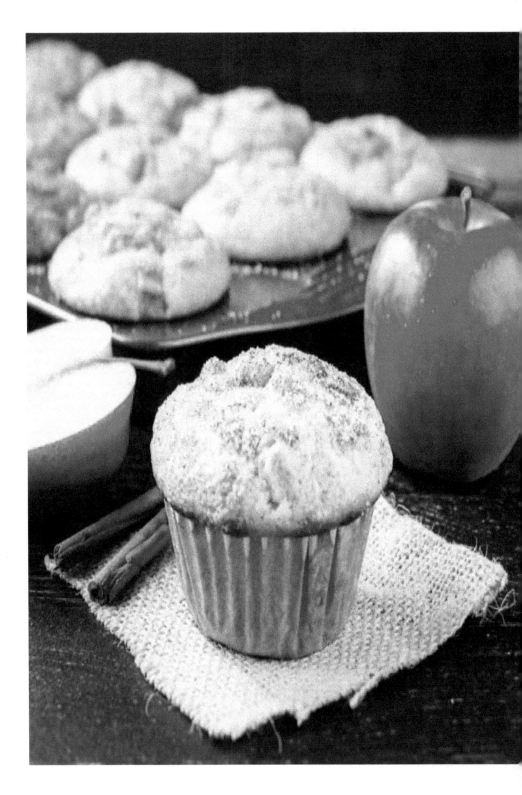

Table of Contents

INTRODUCTION

A plant-based diet is a diet consisting mostly or entirely of plant-based foods with no animal products or artificial ingredients. While a plant-based diet avoids or has limited animal products, it is not necessarily vegan. This includes not only fruits and vegetables, but also nuts, seeds, oils, whole grains, legumes, and beans. It doesn't mean that you are vegetarian or vegan and never eat meat, eggs, or dairy.

Vegetarian diets have also been shown to support health, including a lower risk of developing coronary heart disease, high blood pressure, diabetes, and increased longevity.

Plant-based diets offer all the necessary carbohydrates, vitamins, protein, fats, and minerals for optimal health, and are often higher in fiber and phytonutrients. However, some vegans may need to add a supplement to ensure they receive all the nutrients required.

Who says that plant-based diets are limited or boring? There are lots of delicious recipes that you can use to make mouthwatering, healthy, plant-based dishes that will satisfy your cravings. If you're eating these plant-based foods regularly, you can maintain a healthy weight without obsessing about calories and avoid diseases that result from bad dietary habits.

Benefits of a Plant-Based Diet

Eating a plant-based diet improves the health of your gut so you are better able to absorb the nutrients from food that support your immune system and reduce inflammation. Fiber can lower cholesterol and stabilize blood sugar, and it's great for good bowel management.

- **A Plant-Based Diet May Lower Your Blood Pressure**
  High blood pressure, or hypertension, can increase the risk for health issues, including heart disease, stroke, and type 2 diabetes and reduce blood pressure and other risky conditions.

- **A Plant-Based Diet May Keep Your Heart Healthy**
  Saturated fat in meat can contribute to heart issues when eaten in excess, so plant-based foods can help keep your heart healthy.

- **A Plant-Based Diet May Help Prevent Type 2 Diabetes**
  Animal foods can increase cholesterol levels, so eating a plant-based diet filled with high-quality plant foods can reduce the risk of developing type 2 diabetes by 34 percent.

- **Eating a Plant-Based Diet Could Help You Lose Weight**
  Cutting back on meat can help you to maintain a healthy weight because a plant-based diet is naturally satisfying and rich in fiber.

- **Following a Plant-Based Diet Long Term May Help You Live Longer**
  If you stick with healthy plant-based foods your whole body will be leaner and healthier, allowing you to stay healthy and vital as you age.

- **A Plant-Based Diet May Decrease Your Risk of Cancer**
  Vegetarians have an 18 percent lower risk of cancer compared to non-vegetarians. This is because a plant-based diet is rich of fibers and healthy nutrients.

- **A Plant-Based Diet May Improve Your Cholesterol**
  High cholesterol can lead to fatty deposits in the blood, which can restrict blood flow and potentially lead to heart attack, stroke, heart disease, and many other problems. A plant-based diet can help in maintaining healthy cholesterol levels.

- **Ramping Up Your Plant Intake May Keep Your Brain Strong**
  Increased consumption of fruits and vegetables is associated with a 20 percent reduction in the risk of cognitive impairment and dementia. So plant foods can help protect your brain from multiple issues.

What to Eat in Plant-Based Diets

Fruits: Berries, citrus fruits, pears, peaches, pineapple, bananas, etc.

Vegetables: Kale, spinach, tomatoes, broccoli, cauliflower, carrots, asparagus, peppers, etc.

Starchy vegetables: Potatoes, sweet potatoes, butternut squash, etc.

Whole grains: Brown rice, rolled oats, farro, quinoa, brown rice pasta, barley, etc.

Healthy fats: Avocados, olive oil, coconut oil, unsweetened coconut, etc.

Legumes: Peas, chickpeas, lentils, peanuts, black beans, etc.

Seeds, nuts, and nut butters: Almonds, cashews, macadamia nuts, pumpkin seeds, sunflower seeds, natural peanut butter, tahini, etc.

Unsweetened plant-based milks: Coconut milk, almond milk, cashew milk, etc.

Spices, herbs, and seasonings: Basil, rosemary, turmeric, curry, black pepper, salt, etc.

Condiments: Salsa, mustard, nutritional yeast, soy sauce, vinegar, lemon juice, etc.

Plant-based protein: Tofu, tempeh, plant-based protein sources or powders with no added sugar or artificial ingredients.

Beverages: Coffee, tea, sparkling water, etc.

What Not to Eat in Plant-Based Diets

Fast food: French fries, cheeseburgers, hot dogs, chicken nuggets, etc.

Added sugars and sweets: Table sugar, soda, juice, pastries, cookies, candy, sweet tea, sugary cereals, etc.

Refined grains: White rice, white pasta, white bread, bagels, etc.

Packaged and convenience foods: Chips, crackers, cereal bars, frozen dinners, etc.

Processed vegan-friendly foods: Plant-based meats like; Tofurkey, faux cheeses, vegan butters, etc.

Artificial sweeteners: Equal, Splenda, Sweet'N Low, etc.

Processed animal products: Bacon, lunch meats, sausage, beef jerky, etc.

Day 1:

Breakfast (304 calories)

- 1 serving Berry-Kefir Smoothie

A.M. Snack (95 calories)

- 1 medium apple

Lunch (374 calories)

- 1 serving Green Salad with Pita Bread & Hummus

P.M. Snack (206 calories)

- 1/4 cup dry-roasted unsalted almonds

Dinner (509 calories)

- 1 serving Beefless Vegan Tacos
- 2 cups mixed greens
- 1 serving Citrus Vinaigrette

Day 2:

Breakfast (258 calories)

- 1 serving Cinnamon Roll Overnight Oats
- 1 medium orange

A.M. Snack (341 calories)

- 1 cup low-fat plain Greek yogurt
- 1 medium peach
- 3 Tbsps slivered almonds

Lunch (332 calories)

- 1 serving Thai-Style Chopped Salad with Sriracha Tofu

P.M. Snack (131 calories)

- 1 large pear

Dinner (458 calories)

- 1 serving Mexican Quinoa Salad

Day 3:

Breakfast (258 calories)

- 1 serving Cinnamon Roll Overnight Oats
- 1 medium orange

A.M. Snack (95 calories)

- 1 medium apple

Lunch (463 calories)

- 1 serving Thai-Style Chopped Salad with Sriracha Tofu
- 1 large pear

P.M. Snack (274 calories)

- 1/3 cup dried walnut halves
- 1 medium peach

Dinner (419 calories)

- 1 serving Eggs in Tomato Sauce with Chickpeas & Spinach
- 1 1-oz. slice whole-wheat baguette

BREAKFAST

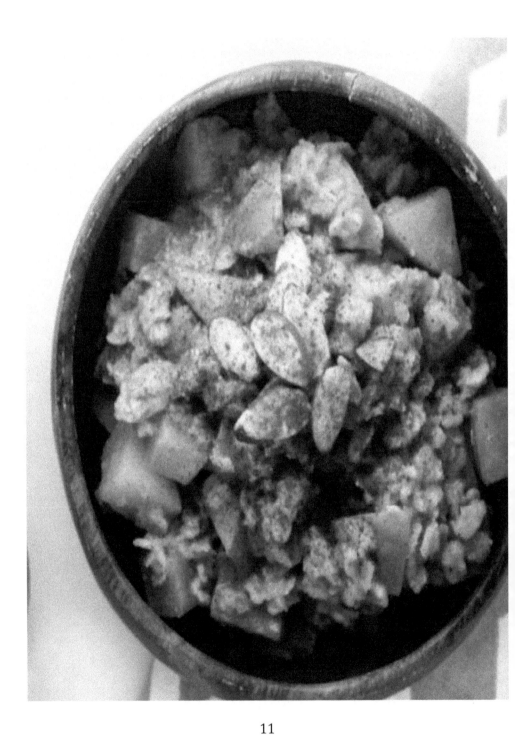

Servings: 4

Preparation Time: 20 minutes

Ingredients:

- 2 pears, peeled, cored, and chopped
- 2 1/2 cups apple cider
- 2 tbsps pure date syrup
- 1 1/3 cup rolled oats
- 2 tsps ground cinnamon

Procedure:

1. First, pour the apple cider in a pot over medium heat and bring it to a boil.
2. Now, add in the pear, oats, and cinnamon.
3. Then, lower the heat and simmer for 3-4 minutes, until the oatmeal thickens.
4. After, that divide between bowls and drizzle with date syrup.
5. Finally, serve immediately.

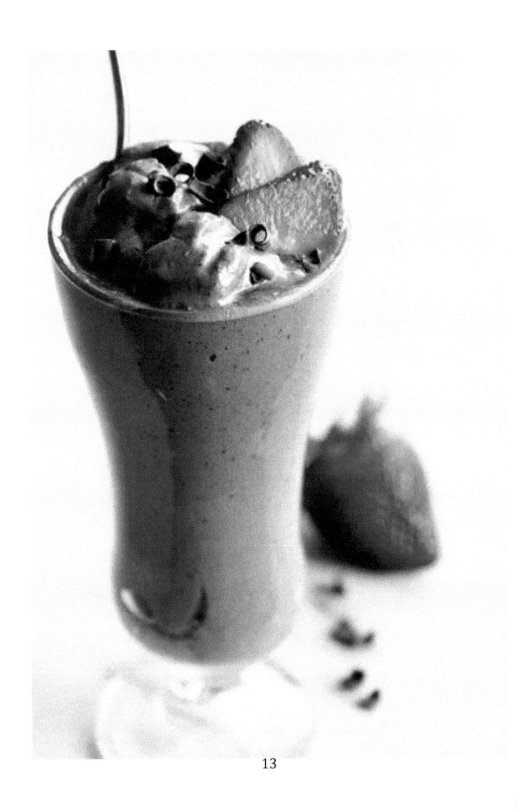

Servings: 4

Preparation Time: 10 minutes

Ingredients:

- 4 cups unsweetened soy milk
- 4 tbsps cocoa powder
- 2 tbsps poppy seeds
- 4 cups blackberries
- 4 tbsps pure agave syrup

Procedure:

1. Submerge poppy seeds in soy milk and let sit for 5 minutes.
2. Then, transfer to a food processor and add in the soy milk, blackberries, agave syrup, and cocoa powder.
3. Now, blitz until smooth.
4. Then, serve right away in glasses.

Servings: 8

Preparation Time: 30 minutes

Per Serving: Calories: 198; Fat: 9.4g; Carbs: 24.5g; Protein: 5.2g

Ingredients:

- 2 teaspoons baking powder
- 1/2 teaspoon Himalayan salt
- 1 cup whole-wheat white flour
- 2 teaspoons sugar
- 1 cup oat flour
- 1 teaspoon ground allspice
- 1 teaspoon ground cinnamon
- 4 tablespoons coconut oil
- 1 cup pumpkin puree
- 1 teaspoon crystalized ginger
- 2 teaspoons lemon juice, freshly squeezed
- 1 cup almond milk

Procedure:

1. Take a mixing bowl, thoroughly combine the flour, baking powder, salt, sugar, and spices.
2. Gradually add in the lemon juice, milk, and pumpkin puree.
3. Now, heat an electric griddle on medium and lightly slick it with coconut oil.

4. Then, cook your cake for approximately 3 minutes until the bubbles form; flip it and cook on the other side for 3 minutes longer until browned on the underside.
5. Repeat with the remaining oil and batter.
6. Finally, serve dusted with cinnamon sugar, if desired.

Servings: 8

Preparation Time: 15 minutes

Per Serving: Calories: 452; Fat: 24.3g; Carbs: 38g; Protein: 25.6g

Ingredients:

- 2 tablespoons nutritional yeast
- 32 ounces extra-firm tofu
- 1/2 teaspoon turmeric powder
- 4 tablespoons olive oil
- 4 handfuls fresh kale, chopped
- 8 slices vegan cheese
- 8 tablespoons ketchup
- Kosher salt and ground black pepper, to taste
- 8 English muffins, cut in half

Procedure:

1. First, heat the olive oil in a frying skillet over medium heat.
2. When it's hot, add the tofu and sauté for 8 minutes, occasionally stirring to promote even cooking.
3. Then, add in the nutritional yeast, turmeric, and kale and continue sautéing for an additional 2 minutes or until the kale wilts.
4. Now, season with salt and pepper to taste.

5. Meanwhile, toast the English muffins until crisp.
6. To assemble the sandwiches, spread the bottom halves of the English muffins with ketchup; top them with the tofu mixture and vegan cheese; place the bun topper on, close the sandwiches and serve warm.

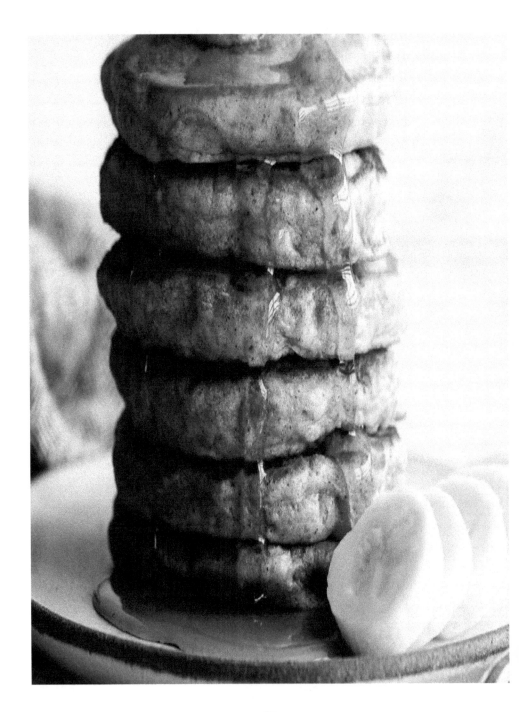

Servings: 8

Preparation Time: 25 minutes

Per Serving: Calories: 302; Fat: 15g; Carbs: 37.2g; Protein: 7.1g

Ingredients:

- 1 cup coconut flour
- 1 cup oat flour
- 4 tablespoons ground flaxseeds
- 1 cup instant oats
- 2 teaspoons baking powder
- 1/2 teaspoon kosher salt
- 1/2 teaspoon ground cardamom
- 1/2 teaspoon ground cinnamon
- 2 cups banana
- 4 tablespoons coconut oil, at room temperature
- 1 teaspoon coconut extract

Procedure:

1. To make the "flax" egg, in a small mixing dish, whisk 2 tablespoons of the ground flaxseeds with 4 tablespoons of water.
2. Now, let it sit for at least 15 minutes.
3. Take a mixing bowl, thoroughly combine the flour, oats, baking powder, and spices.
4. Now, add in the flax egg and mashed banana.

5. Then, mix until everything is well incorporated.
6. After, that heat 1/2 tablespoon of the coconut oil in a frying pan over medium-low flame.
7. Now, spoon about 1/4 cup of the batter into the frying pan; fry your pancake for approximately 3 minutes per side.
8. Then, repeat until you run out of batter.
9. Lastly, serve with your favorite fixings and enjoy!

Servings: 4

Preparation Time: 20 minutes

Per Serving: Calories: 233; Fat: 6.5g; Carbs: 35.5g; Protein: 8.2g

Ingredients:

- 2 tablespoons ground flax seeds
- A pinch of sea salt
- 1 teaspoon vanilla paste
- A pinch of grated nutmeg
- 8 slices bread
- 2 cups coconut milk
- 2 tablespoons agave syrup
- 1 teaspoon ground cinnamon
- 1/2 teaspoon ground cloves

Procedure:

1. Take a mixing bowl, thoroughly combine the flax seeds, coconut milk, vanilla, salt, nutmeg, cinnamon, cloves, and agave syrup.
2. Dredge each slice of bread into the milk mixture until well coated on all sides.

3. Now, preheat an electric griddle to medium heat and lightly oil it with a non-stick cooking spray.
4. Then, cook each slice of bread on the preheated griddle for about 3 minutes per side until golden brown.
5. Bon appétit

Servings: 18

Preparation Time: 30 minutes

Per Serving: Calories: 258; Fat: 10.7g; Carbs: 37.8g;
Protein: 3.1g

Ingredients:

- 4 tablespoons maple syrup
- 1 cup brown sugar
- 3 cups all-purpose flour
- 4 ripe bananas
- 1 teaspoon baking powder
- 1 cup pecans, chopped
- 8 tablespoons coconut oil, room temperature
- 1/2 teaspoon ground cardamom
- 2/3 teaspoon ground cinnamon
- 1 teaspoon baking soda
- 1 teaspoon salt
- 1/2 teaspoon grated nutmeg

Procedure:

1. Begin by preheating your oven to 350 degrees F.
   Coat 18-cup muffin tin with muffin liners.
2. Take a mixing bowl, mash the bananas; stir in the
   coconut oil, maple syrup, and sugar.

3. Gradually stir in the flour, followed by the baking powder, baking soda, and spices.
4. Now, stir to combine well and fold in the pecans.
5. Then, scrape the mixture into the prepared muffin tin.
6. Finally, bake your muffins in the preheated oven for about 27 minutes or until a tester comes out dry and clean. Bon appétit!

Servings: 8

Preparation Time: 5-15 minutes

Per Serving: Calories 339 Fats 24. 5g Carbs 30g Protein 2. 3g

Ingredients:

For the berry cream:

- 4 tbsps pure date sugar
- 2 tsps vanilla extract
- 1 cup whipped coconut cream
- 1 cup fresh raspberries
- 1 cup fresh blueberries
- 2 knobs plant butter

For the crepes:

- 2 tsps pure date sugar
- 4 tbsps flax seed powder + 12 tbsps water
- 1/2 tsp salt
- 2 tsps vanilla extract
- 3 cups water
- 6 tbsps plant butter for frying
- 4 cups almond flour
- 3 cups almond milk

Procedure:

1. First, melt butter in a pot over low heat and mix in the date sugar and vanilla.
2. Then, cook until the sugar melts and Then toss in berries.
3. Allow softening for 2 3 minutes.
4. Set aside to cool.
5. Take a medium bowl, mix the flax seed powder with water and allow thickening for 5 minutes to make the flax egg.
6. Whisk in the vanilla, date sugar, and salt.
7. Now, pour in a quarter cup of almond flour and whisk; then, a quarter cup of almond milk, and mix until no lumps remain.
8. Then, repeat the mixing process with the remaining almond flour and almond milk in the same quantities until exhausted.
9. Now, mix in 1 cup of water until the mixture is runny like that of pancakes, and add the remaining water until the mixture is lighter.
10. Brush a large non-stick skillet with some butter and place over medium heat to melt.
11. After, that pour 1 tablespoon of the batter into the pan and swirl the skillet quickly and all around to coat the pan with the batter.
12. Now, cook until the batter is dry and golden brown beneath, about 30 seconds.
13. Use a spatula to carefully flip the crepe and cook the other side until golden brown too.

14. Then, fold the crepe onto a plate and set it aside.
15. Repeat making more crepes with the remaining batter until exhausted.
16. Plate the crepes, top with the whipped coconut cream, and the berry compote.
17. Lastly, serve immediately

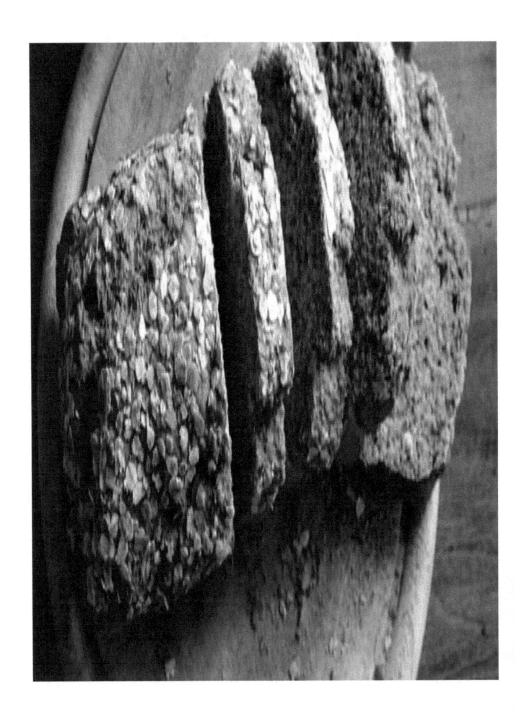

Servings: 8

Preparation Time: 5-15 minutes

Per Serving: Calories 963 Fats 44. 4g Carbs 125. 1g Protein 22. 1g

Ingredients:

- 1 cup rolled oats
- 4 tbsps pure maple syrup
- 8 cups whole-wheat flour
- 1/2 tsp salt
- 2 tsps baking soda
- 2 1/3 cups coconut milk, thick

Procedure:

1. First, preheat the oven to 400 F.
2. Take a bowl, mix flour, salt, oats, and baking soda.
3. Now, add in coconut milk, maple syrup, and whisk until dough forms.
4. Dust your hands with some flour and knead the dough into a ball.
5. Then, shape the dough into a circle and place it on a baking sheet.

6. After, that cut a deep cross on the dough and bake in the oven for 15 minutes at 450 F.
7. Then, reduce the temperature to 400 F and bake further for 20 to 25 minutes or until a hollow sound is made when the bottom of the bread is tapped.
8. In the end, slice and serve.

Servings: 8

Preparation Time: 5-15 minutes

Per Serving: Calories 1133 Fats 74. 9g Carbs 104. 3g Protein 18g

Ingredients:

For the muffins:

- 4 apples, peeled, cored, and chopped
- 1 1/3 cups pure date sugar
- 2 flax seed powder + 6 tbsps water
- 4 tsps baking powder
- 1/2 tsp salt
- 2/3 cup flax milk
- 3 cups whole-wheat flour
- 2 tsps cinnamon powder
- 2/3 cup melted plant butter

For topping:

- 3 tsps cinnamon powder
- 1 cup pure date sugar
- 1 cup cold plant butter, cubed
- 2/3 cup whole-wheat flour

Procedure:

1. Preheat the oven to 400 F and grease 6 muffin cups with cooking spray.
2. Take a bowl, mix the flax seed powder with water and allow thickening for 5 minutes to make the flax egg.
3. Then, in a medium bowl, mix the flour, date sugar, baking powder, salt, and cinnamon powder.
4. Whisk in the butter, flax egg, flax milk, and then fold in the apples.
5. Now, fill the muffin cups two-thirds way up with the batter.
6. Take a small bowl, mix the remaining flour, date sugar, cold butter, and cinnamon powder. Sprinkle the mixture on the muffin batter.
7. Bake for 20-minutes.
8. Then, remove the muffins onto a wire rack, allow cooling, and serve warm.

Servings: 8

Preparation Time: 5-15 minutes

Per Serving: Calories 326 Fats 14. 3g Carbs 38. 3g Protein 12. 5g

Ingredients:

- 1/2 cup chopped toasted walnuts
- 4 tbsps pure malt syrup
- 8 cups almond milk Dairy-Free yogurt, cold
- 4 cups mixed berries, halved or chopped

Procedure:

1. Take a medium bowl, mix the yogurt and malt syrup until well-combined.
2. Now, divide the mixture into 4 breakfast bowls.
3. Then, top with the berries and walnuts.
4. Enjoy immediately.

Servings: 8

Preparation Time: 5-15 minutes

Per Serving: Calories 379 Fats 35. 6g Carbs 14. 8g Protein 5. 6g

Ingredients:

- 2 tsps pure date sugar
- 4 tbsps flax seed powder + 12 tbsps water
- 1/2 tsp salt
- 2 tsps vanilla extract
- 6 tbsps fresh orange juice
- 4 cups almond flour
- 6 tbsps plant butter for frying
- 3 cups oat milk
- 1 cup melted plant butter

Procedure:

1. Take a medium bowl, mix the flax seed powder with 1 cup water and allow thickening for 5 minutes to make the flax egg.
2. Whisk in the vanilla, date sugar, and salt.
3. Now, pour in a quarter cup of almond flour and whisk, then a quarter cup of oat milk, and mix until no lumps remain.

4. Repeat the mixing process with the remaining almond flour and almond milk in the same quantities until exhausted.
5. Then, mix in the plant butter, orange juice, and half of the water until the mixture is runny like that of pancakes.
6. After, add the remaining water until the mixture is lighter.
7. Brush a large non-stick skillet with some butter and place over medium heat to melt.
8. Then, pour 1 tablespoon of the batter into the pan and swirl the skillet quickly and all around to coat the pan with the batter.
9. Now, cook until the batter is dry and golden brown beneath, about 30 seconds.
10. Use a spatula to carefully flip the crepe and cook the other side until golden brown too.
11. After, that fold the crepe onto a plate and set it aside.
12. Repeat making more crepes with the remaining batter until exhausted.
13. In the end, drizzle some maple syrup on the crepes and serve.

SALADS

Servings: 8

Preparation Time: 10 minutes

Ingredients:

- 2 cups fresh blackberries
- 1 1/2 cups olive oil
- 1/2 red onion, thinly sliced
- 2 cups raisins
- 20 oz. baby spinach
- Sea salt and black pepper to taste
- 1 cup chopped pecans
- 1/2 cup balsamic vinegar

Procedure:

1. First, combine the spinach, raisins, blackberries, red onion, and pecans in a bowl.
2. Take another bowl, mix the vinegar, olive oil, salt, and pepper.
3. Now, pour over the salad and toss to coat.
4. Lastly, serve immediately.

Servings: 8

Preparation Time: 25 minutes

Ingredients:

- 2 cups firm tofu, drained and cubed
- 4 tbsps minced fresh parsley
- Black pepper to taste
- 4 tbsps white wine vinegar
- 3 lbs small potatoes, unpeeled
- 2 tbsps minced fresh chives
- 2 tsps minced fresh tarragon
- 2/3 cup olive oil

Procedure:

1. First, place the potatoes in a pot with boiling salted water and cook for 20 minutes.
2. Drain, cool, and slice.
3. Now, remove it to a bowl.
4. Then, stir in tofu, parsley, chives, and tarragon.
5. Take another bowl, mix the oil, vinegar, and pepper.
6. Then, pour over the salad and toss to coat.
7. In the end, let it chill and serve.

Special Mom's Cauliflower Coleslaw

Servings: 8

Preparation Time: 10 minutes + chilling time

Per Serving: Calories: 280; Fat: 24.6g; Carbs: 13.8g; Protein: 3.3g

Ingredients:

- 2 cups carrots, trimmed and shredded
- 4 cups small cauliflower florets, frozen and thawed
- 2 medium onions, chopped
- 4 cups red cabbage, shredded
- 1 cup vegan mayonnaise
- 1 teaspoon cayenne pepper
- 8 tablespoons coconut yogurt, unsweetened
- Sea salt and ground black pepper, to taste
- 2 tablespoons yellow mustard
- 2 tablespoons fresh lemon juice

Procedure:

1. Take a salad bowl, toss the vegetables until well combined.
2. Take a small mixing bowl, thoroughly combine the remaining ingredients.
3. Then, add the mayo dressing to the vegetables and toss to combine well.
4. Now, place the coleslaw in your refrigerator until ready to serve. Bon appétit!

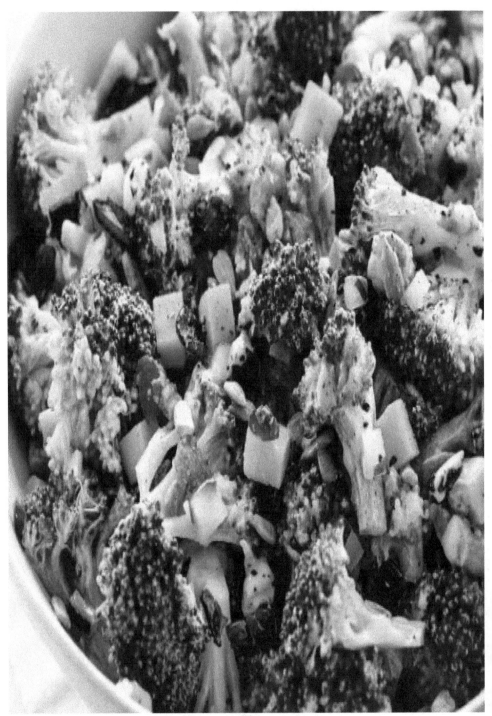

Servings: 8

Preparation Time: 10 minutes + chilling time

Per Serving: Calories: 417; Fat: 30.6g; Carbs: 28.3g; Protein: 13.7g

Ingredients:

- 1/2 cup pine nuts
- 4 pounds broccoli florets
- 2 teaspoons mustard
- 2 shallots, chopped
- 4 garlic cloves, finely chopped
- 2 cups vegan mayonnaise
- 1/2 cup sunflower seeds
- Sea salt and freshly ground black pepper, to taste
- 1 cup pomegranate seeds
- 2 tablespoons balsamic vinegar
- 2 tablespoons fresh lime juice

Procedure:

1. Take a saucepan, bring about 1/4 inch of water to a boil.
2. Now, add in the broccoli florets.
3. Then, cover and steam the broccoli until crisp-tender or about 5 minutes.
4. Now, let the broccoli florets cool completely and place them in a salad bowl.

5. After, add in the sunflower seeds, pine nuts, shallot, garlic, mayo, balsamic vinegar, lime juice, mustard, salt, and black pepper.
6. Then, toss to combine well.
7. Finally, garnish with pomegranate seeds and serve well-chilled. Bon appétit!

Delicious Creamed Cavatappi and Cauliflower Salad

Servings: 8

Preparation Time: 15 minutes + chilling time

Per Serving: Calories: 523; Fat: 22.2g; Carbs: 69g; Protein: 12.6g

Ingredients:

- 1 cup vegan mayonnaise
- 2 tablespoons fresh lemon juice
- 24 ounces Cavatappi pasta
- 4 medium tomatoes, sliced
- 2 onions, chopped
- 2 cups cauliflower florets
- 4 cups arugula, torn into pieces
- 4 garlic cloves, finely chopped
- 2 teaspoons deli mustard

Procedure:

1. First, bring a large pot of salted water to a boil.
2. Now, cook the pasta and cauliflower florets for about 6 minutes.
3. Then, remove the cauliflower with a slotted spoon from the water.
4. Now, continue to cook your pasta for a further 6 minutes until al dente.

5. Allow the pasta and cauliflower to cool completely; then, transfer them to a salad bowl.
6. Then, add in the remaining ingredients and toss until well combined.
7. In the end, taste and adjust the seasonings; place the salad in your refrigerator until ready to use. Bon appétit!

Servings: 10

Preparation Time: 10 minutes + chilling time

Per Serving: Calories: 338; Fat: 16.3g; Carbs: 37.2g;
Protein: 13g

Ingredients:

- 3 pounds French green beans, trimmed
- 2 white onions, thinly sliced
- 4 garlic cloves, minced
- Himalayan salt and ground black pepper, to taste
- 1/2 cup extra-virgin olive oil
- 4 tablespoons fresh lime juice
- 4 tablespoons tamari sauce
- 2 tablespoons mustard
- 4 tablespoons sesame seeds, lightly toasted
- 4 tablespoons fresh mint leaves, roughly chopped

Procedure:

1. First, boil the green beans in a large saucepan of salted water until they are just tender or about 2 minutes.
2. Drain and let the beans cool completely; Then, transfer them to a salad bowl.

3. Then, add in the onion, garlic, salt, black pepper, olive oil, lime juice, tamari sauce, and mustard.
4. Now, top your salad with sesame seeds and mint leaves.
5. Bon appétit!

Servings: 8

Preparation Time: 15 minutes

Per Serving: Calories: 559; Fat: 20.3g; Carbs: 85.5g; Protein: 15.3g

Ingredients:

- 8 tablespoons dry white wine
- 24 ounces shell pasta
- 4 Roma tomatoes, diced
- 2 cups radicchio, sliced
- 2 teaspoons Italian seasoning blend
- 2 pounds eggplants, cut into rounds
- 1 teaspoon lemon zest
- 2 tablespoons olive oil
- Sea salt and ground black pepper, to taste
- 1 cup olives, pitted and halved
- 8 tablespoons extra-virgin olive oil
- 4 tablespoons balsamic vinegar

Procedure:

1. First, heat 2 tablespoons of olive oil in a cast-iron skillet over a moderate flame.
2. Once hot, fry the eggplant for about 10 minutes until browned on all sides.
3. Meanwhile, cook the pasta according to the package directions.

4. Now, drain and rinse the pasta.
5. Let it cool completely and then, transfer it to a salad bowl.
6. Then, add in the remaining ingredients, including the cooked eggplant; toss until well combined.

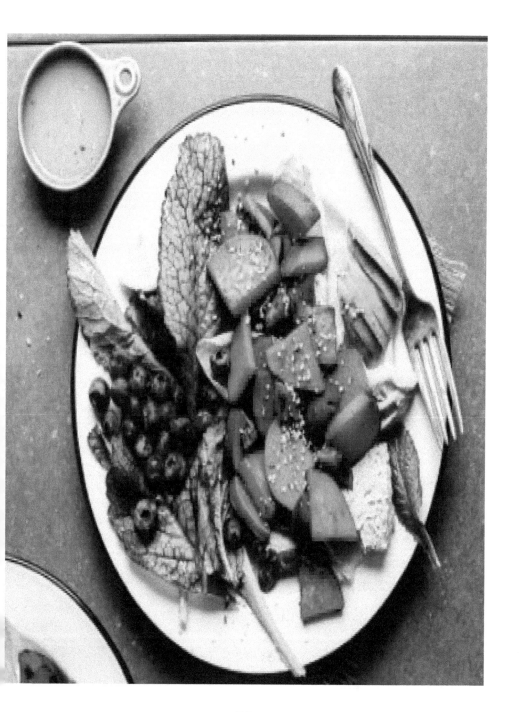

Servings: 4

Preparation Time: 15-30 minutes

Per Serving: Carbs: 57. 6g Protein: 7. 5g Fats: 37. 6g Calories: 523 Kcal

Ingredients:

For the sweet potatoes:

- 2 tbsps coconut oil
- 2 pinch salt and pepper
- 4 small potatoes

For the Dressing:

- 6 tbsps lemon juice
- 2 pinches of salt and pepper
- 2 tbsps extra virgin olive oil

For the Salad:

- 6 tbsps lemon juice
- 2 pinch salt and pepper
- 8 cups mixed greens
- 2 tbsps extra virgin olive oil

For Servings:

- 4 tbsps hemp seeds
- 2 cups blueberries

- 2 medium ripe avocadoes
- 8 tbsps hummus
- Fresh chopped parsley

Procedure:

1. Take a large skillet and apply gentle heat
2. Now, add sweet potatoes, coat them with salt and pepper, and pour some oil
3. Then, cook till sweet potatoes turn browns
4. Take a bowl and mix lemon juice, salt, and pepper
5. After, add salad, sweet potatoes, and the serving together
6. Finally, mix well and dress and serve

Special Balsamic Beans Salad

Servings: 8

Preparation Time: 10 minutes

Per Serving: Calories145, Total Fat 10.9g, Saturated Fat 2.6g, Cholesterol 14mg, Sodium 263mg, Total Carbohydrate 9.4g, Dietary Fiber 1.5g, Total Sugars 3.1g, Protein 3.3g, Calcium 67mg, Iron 1mg, Potassium 94mg, Phosphorus 44mg

Ingredients:

- Black pepper to taste
- 1 cup chopped green onions
- 2 cups of frozen green beans
- 1/2 cup chopped almonds
- 1 1/2 cups mayonnaise
- 4 tablespoons balsamic vinegar

Procedure:

1. First, place beans in a colander, and run warm water over them until they are thawed.
2. Place in a large bowl.
3. Now, toast almonds in a skillet over medium heat.
4. Then, combine with beans.
5. Now, stir in onions and mayonnaise.
6. Then, mix in balsamic vinegar and season with pepper.
7. Cover, and refrigerate.

Servings: 8

Preparation Time: 10 minutes

Per Serving: Calories 76, Total Fat 5g, Saturated Fat 1.2g, Cholesterol 2mg, Sodium 131mg, Total Carbohydrate 5.9g, Dietary Fiber 1.3g, Total Sugars 2.8g, Protein 1.8g, Calcium 59mg, Iron 1mg, Potassium 146mg, Phosphorus 88mg

Ingredients:

- 2 teaspoons honey
- 1/4 teaspoon salt
- 1 cup dried cranberries
- 1 cup roasted cauliflower
- 2 tablespoons olive oil
- 1/2 teaspoon ground black pepper
- 1 cup lemon juice
- 2 bunches of kale, cut into bite-size pieces

Procedure:

1. First, whisk lemon juice, olive oil, honey, salt, and black pepper in a large bowl.
2. Now, add kale, cauliflower, and cranberries; toss to combine.

Servings: 8

Preparation Time: 5 minutes

Per Serving: Calories 80, Total Fat 2.9g, Saturated Fat 0.4g, Cholesterol 0mg, Sodium 115mg, Total Carbohydrate 13g, Dietary Fiber 1.1g, Total Sugars 5.6g, Protein 2g, Calcium 78mg, Iron 1mg, Potassium 231mg, Phosphorus156mg

Ingredients:

- 4 tablespoons water
- 4 tablespoons olive oil
- 6 tablespoons lemon juice
- 16 cups thinly sliced kale, packed
- 2 tablespoons minced garlic
- 2 cucumbers, peeled and sliced
- 2 tablespoons soy sauce
- 4 teaspoons honey

Procedure:

1. First, combine olive oil, lemon juice, water, garlic, soy sauce, and honey in a small bowl.
2. Now, stir until smooth.
3. Then, place kale and cucumbers in a large bowl.
4. After, pour dressing over kale; toss until combined.
5. Marinate for a minimum of 20 minutes, tossing occasionally.
6. Finally, serve.

Servings: 8

Preparation Time: 10 minutes

Per Serving: Calories: 140 Cal Fat: 8 g Carbs: 8 g Protein: 10 g Fiber: 4 g

Ingredients:

For the Meatballs:

- 1 cup quinoa, cooked
- 2 cups cooked black beans
- 6 cloves of garlic, peeled
- 2 small red onions, peeled
- 2 teaspoons ground dried coriander
- 2 teaspoons ground dried cumin
- 2 teaspoons smoked paprika

For the Salad:

- 2 large sweet potatoes, peeled, diced
- 2 lemons, juiced
- 2 teaspoons minced garlic
- 2 cups coriander leaves
- 2/3 cup almonds
- 2/3 teaspoon ground black pepper
- 1 teaspoon salt
- 3 tablespoons olive oil

Procedure:

1. First, prepare the meatballs and for this, place beans and puree in a blender, pulse until pureed, and place this mixture in a medium bowl.
2. Now, add onion and garlic, process until chopped, add to the bean mixture, add all the spices, stir until combined, and shape the mixture into uniform balls.
3. Then, bake the balls on a greased baking sheet for 25 minutes at 350 degrees F until browned.
4. Meanwhile, spread sweet potatoes on a baking sheet lined with baking paper, drizzle with ½ tablespoon oil, toss until coated, then bake for 20 minutes with the meatballs.
5. Prepare the dressing, and for this, place the remaining ingredients for the salad in a food processor and pulse until smooth.
6. After, place roasted sweet potatoes in a bowl, drizzle with the dressing, toss until coated, and then top with meatballs.
7. Finally, serve straight away.

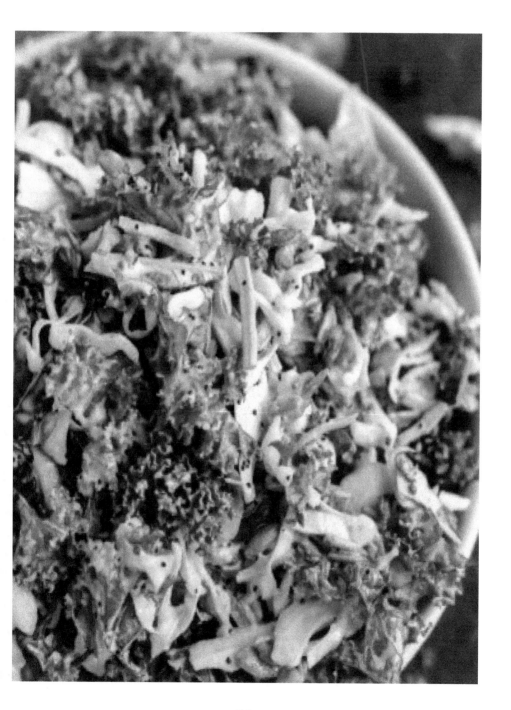

Servings: 8

Preparation Time: 10-75 minutes

Per Serving: Calories: 140 Cal Fat: 0.9 g Carbs: 27.1 g
Protein: 6.3 g Fiber: 6.2 g

Ingredients:

- 1/2 onion, thinly sliced
- 1 small head cabbage, shredded
- 2 small bunches of kale, chopped
- salt, pepper, and chili flakes
- 4 garlic cloves, minced
- 1/2 cup tender herbs (cilantro, basil, parsley, chives)
- 1/2 cup olive oil
- 8 tablespoons lemon juice

Procedure:

1. First, combine kale, cabbage, herbs, and onions in a large bowl.
2. Now, add olive oil, lemon juice, minced garlic, salt, pepper, and mix well.
3. Then, add chili flakes, toss well before serving.

MAIN DISHES

Easy Sweet Potatoes

Servings: 8

Preparation Time: 29 minutes

Per Serving: Calories: 140 Cal Fat: 0.9 g Carbs: 27.1 g Protein: 6.3 g Fiber: 6.2 g

Ingredients:

- 3 cups water
- 8 sweet potatoes, scrubbed and rinsed
- Optional toppings:
- Arugula, olive oil, lemon, sea salt
- Scrambled tofu, avocado, tomatoes
- Vegan butter, coconut sugar, cinnamon

Procedure:

1. Start by adding water to the instant pot.
2. Now, place the steaming tray inside and put potatoes on top.
3. Then, cover with lid and seal.
4. Pressure cook for 18 minutes in manual mode.
5. When done cooking, allow pressure to release on its own (about 15 minutes).
6. Now, remove the lid.
7. Lastly, serve immediately with desired toppings. Enjoy!

Servings: 12

Preparation Time: 40 minutes

Ingredients:

- 4 tbsps nutritional yeast
- 4 tsps paprika
- 2 tsps cayenne pepper
- Salt to taste
- 2 cups shredded watercress
- 16 small corn tortillas, warm
- 4 tbsps whole-wheat flour
- 2 limes, cut into wedges
- 2 heads cauliflower, cut into pieces
- 4 tbsps olive oil
- 4 cups cherry tomatoes, halved
- 4 carrots, grated
- 1 cup mango salsa
- 1 cup guacamole

Procedure:

1. Preheat oven to 350 F.
2. Now, brush the cauliflower with oil in a bowl.
3. Take another bowl, mix the flour, yeast, paprika, cayenne pepper, and salt.
4. Now, pour into the cauliflower bowl and toss to coat.

5. Then, spread the cauliflower on a greased baking sheet.
6. Bake for 20-30 minutes.
7. Take a bowl, combine the watercress, cherry tomatoes, carrots, mango salsa, and guacamole.
8. Once the cauliflower is ready, divide it between the tortillas, add the mango mixture, roll up and serve with lime wedges on the side.

Servings: 8

Preparation Time: 35 minutes

Ingredients:

- 3 tsps ground cumin
- 4 tbsps olive oil
- 4 tsps ground chipotle pepper
- 2 cups black-eyed peas, soaked overnight
- 1 1/2 tsps garlic powder
- 1 tsp smoked paprika
- 1/2 cup sun-dried tomatoes, chopped
- 3 tsps onion powder
- 2 tsps dried oregano

Procedure:

1. First, place the black-eyed peas in a pot and add 2 cups of water, olive oil, chipotle pepper, cumin, onion powder, oregano, garlic powder, salt, and paprika.
2. Now, cook for 20 minutes over medium heat.
3. Then, mix in sun-dried tomatoes, let sit for a few minutes and serve.

Servings: 8

Preparation Time: 25 minutes

Per Serving: Calories: 365; Fat: 23.8g; Carbs: 35.3g; Protein: 6.1g

Ingredients:

- Sea salt and ground black pepper, to taste
- 8 tablespoons olive oil
- 5 pounds carrots washed, trimmed, and halved lengthwise

Sauce:

- 4 tablespoons white vinegar
- 1 teaspoon cumin seed
- 2 teaspoons garlic, pressed
- 4 tablespoons soy sauce
- 2 teaspoons deli mustard
- 2 teaspoons agave syrup
- 8 tablespoons tahini
- 1 teaspoon dried dill weed

Procedure:

1. Begin by preheating your oven to 400 degrees F.
2. Then, toss the carrots with olive oil, salt, and black pepper.

3. Arrange them in a single layer on a parchment-lined roasting sheet.
4. Now, roast the carrots in the preheated oven for about 20 minutes, until crisp-tender.
5. Meanwhile, whisk all the sauce ingredients until well combined.
6. Finally, serve the carrots with the sauce for dipping. Bon appétit!

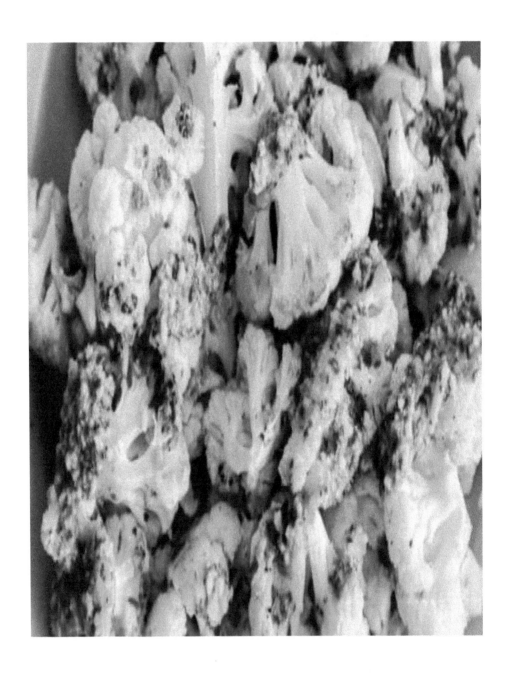

Servings: 8

Preparation Time: 30 minutes

Per Serving: Calories: 175; Fat: 14g; Carbs: 10.7g; Protein: 3.7g

Ingredients:

- 5 pounds cauliflower florets
- 2 tablespoons fresh basil
- 1/2 cup olive oil
- 2 tablespoons fresh coriander
- 2 teaspoons red pepper flakes
- Sea salt and ground black pepper, to taste
- 2 tablespoons fresh oregano
- 8 cloves garlic, whole
- 2 tablespoons fresh rosemary
- 2 tablespoons fresh parsley

Procedure:

1. Begin by preheating the oven to 425 degrees F.
2. Now, toss the cauliflower with the olive oil and arrange them on a parchment-lined roasting pan.
3. Then, roast the cauliflower florets for about 20 minutes; toss them with the garlic and spices and continue cooking an additional 10 minutes.
4. Finally, serve warm. Bon appétit!

Healthy Creamy Rosemary Broccoli Mash

Servings: 8

Preparation Time: 15 minutes

Per Serving: Calories: 155; Fat: 9.8g; Carbs: 14.1g; Protein: 5.7g

Ingredients:

- 8 cloves garlic, chopped
- 4 sprigs fresh rosemary, leaves picked and chopped
- 1/2 cup soy milk, unsweetened
- 3 pounds broccoli florets
- 6 tablespoons vegan butter
- Sea salt and red pepper, to taste

Procedure:

1. First, steam the broccoli florets for about 10 minutes; set it aside to cool.
2. Take a saucepan, melt the vegan butter over moderately high heat; Now, sauté the garlic and rosemary for about 1 minute or until they are fragrant.
3. Now, add the broccoli florets to your food processor, followed by the sautéed garlic/rosemary mixture, salt, pepper, and milk.
4. Now, puree until everything is well incorporated.
5. Finally, garnish with some extra fresh herbs, if desired, and serve hot. Bon appétit!

Servings: 8

Preparation Time: 15 minutes

Per Serving: Calories: 169; Fat: 11.1g; Carbs: 14.9g; Protein: 6.3g

Ingredients:

- 6 tablespoons olive oil
- Sea salt and ground black pepper, to taste
- 4 pounds Swiss chard, tough stalks removed, torn into pieces
- 2 red bell peppers, seeded and diced
- 8 garlic cloves, chopped
- 2 shallots, thinly sliced
- 2 cups vegetable broth

Procedure:

1. Take a saucepan, heat the olive oil over medium-high heat.
2. Then, sauté the shallot and pepper for about 3 minutes or until tender.
3. Then, sauté the garlic for about 1 minute until aromatic.
4. Now, add in the broth and Swiss chard and bring to a boil.
5. After, turn the heat to a simmer and continue to cook for 10 minutes longer.
6. Finally, season with salt and black pepper to taste and serve warm. Bon appétit!

Servings: 8

Preparation Time: 10 minutes

Per Serving: Calories: 205; Fat: 11.8g; Carbs: 17.3g; Protein: 7.6g

Ingredients:

- 6 tablespoons olive oil
- 8 tablespoons scallions, chopped
- 1 teaspoon mustard seeds
- Kosher salt and ground black pepper, to taste
- 8 cloves garlic, minced
- 3 pounds kale
- 1 cup dry white wine
- 1 cup water

Procedure:

1. Take a large saucepan, bring the water to a boil. Add in the kale and let it cook until bright, about 3 minutes.
2. Now, drain and squeeze dry.
3. Then, wipe the saucepan with paper towels and preheat the olive oil over moderate heat.
4. Once hot, cook the scallions and garlic for approximately 2 minutes until they are fragrant.

5. After, add in the wine, flowed by the kale, mustard seeds, salt, black pepper; continue to cook, covered, for a further 5 minutes or until heated through.
6. Lastly, ladle into individual bowls and serve hot. Bon appétit!

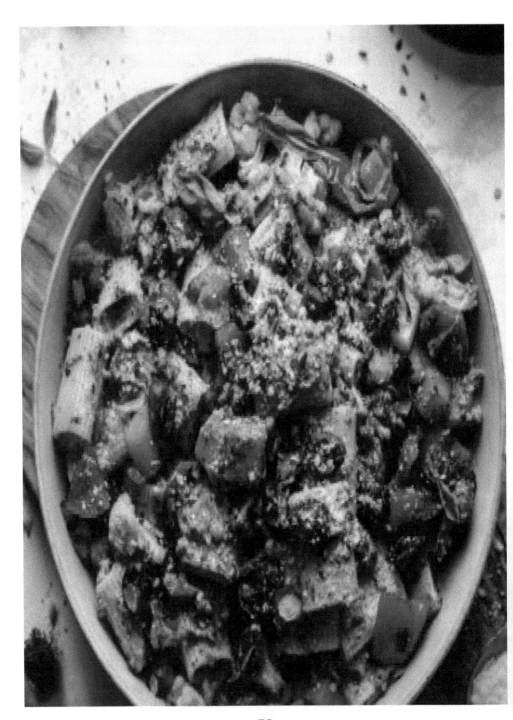

Servings: 4

Preparation Time: 5 minutes

Per Serving: Calories 383, Total Fat 17. 8g, Saturated Fat 10. 1g, Cholesterol 39mg, Sodium 129mg, Total Carbohydrate 44g, Dietary Fiber 2. 4g, Total Sugars 3. 2g, Protein 13. 6g

Ingredients:

- 4 oz. heavy cream
- 8 oz. frozen broccoli florets
- 1/2 cup vegetable broth
- 1 tablespoon coconut oil
- 8 oz. Farfalle pasta
- 1 cup tofu
- 1/2 cup basil pesto

Procedure:

1. Set the Instant Pot; add Farfalline pasta, broccoli, coconut oil, tofu, basil pesto, vegetable broth.
2. Now, cover the Instant Pot and lock it in.
3. Set the Manual or Pressure Cook timer for 10 minutes.
4. Make sure the timer is set to "Sealing".
5. Once the timer reaches zero, quickly release the pressure.
6. Then, add heavy cream.
7. Enjoy.

Servings: 4

Preparation Time: 5 minutes

Per Serving: Calories 509, Total Fat 11.3g, Saturated Fat 6. 4g, Cholesterol 23mg, Sodium 1454mg, Total Carbohydrate 70.3g, Dietary Fiber 10. 8g, Total Sugars 20.5g, Protein 34. 8g

Ingredients:

- 1 teaspoon garlic powder
- 2 small onions
- 1 cup shredded sharp cheddar
- 2 tablespoons coconut flour
- 1 tablespoon chili powder
- 1 tablespoon butter
- 2 cups dry macaroni
- 1/2 teaspoon smoked paprika
- 2 cups cottage cheese
- ½ teaspoon dried basil
- 2 cups tomato paste
- 4 cups vegetable broth

Procedure:

1. First, set the Instant Pot to Sauté.
2. Then, add butter and wait one minute to heat up.
3. Now, add the cottage cheese, sauté for one minute. Stir often.

4. Add coconut flour, onion, and garlic powder.
5. After, add the chili powder, smoked paprika, basil, tomato paste, and 2 cups of vegetable broth. Add the dry macaroni and cottage cheese.
6. Stir well.
7. Then, cover the Instant Pot and lock it in.
8. Set the Manual or Pressure Cook timer for 10 minutes.
9. Make sure the timer is set to "Sealing."
10. Once the timer reaches zero, quickly release the pressure.
11. In the end, add shredded sharp cheddar cheese and enjoy.

Homemade Spicy Cauliflower Pasta

Servings: 4

Preparation Time: 5 minutes

Per Serving: Calories298, Total Fat 10. 4g, Saturated Fat 7.2g, Cholesterol 50mg, Sodium 426mg, Total Carbohydrate 39.6g, Dietary Fiber 1.5g, Total Sugars 1.8g, Protein 12.2g

Ingredients:

- 1/2 teaspoon paprika
- 2 tablespoons coconut oil
- 2 cups vegetable broth
- Salt & pepper to taste
- 2 teaspoons garlic powder
- 1 cup cauliflower florets
- 1 cup broccoli florets
- 2 cups bow tie pasta

Procedure:

1. Set the Instant Pot, set the Sauté button, and add coconut oil when oil is hot; place garlic powder, paprika, cauliflower florets, broccoli florets, salt, and pepper.
2. Sauté the mixture until it's cooked thoroughly.
3. Then, add the vegetable broth and dry bow tie pasta.

4. Now, mix very well and place the lid on the Instant Pot, and bring the toggle switch into the "Sealing" position.
5. Press Manual or Pressure Cook and adjust the time for 5 minutes.
6. When the five minutes are up, do a Natural-release for 5 minutes, and then move the toggle switch to "Venting" to release the rest of the pressure in the pot.
7. Then, remove the lid.
8. If the mixture looks watery, press "Sauté," and bring the mixture up to a boil and let it boil for a few minutes. It will thicken as it boils.
9. Finally, serve and enjoy!

Special n Tasty Mac and Cheese

Servings: 4

Preparation Time: 5 minutes

Per Serving: Calories 210, Total Fat 3g, Saturated Fat 1g, Cholesterol 4mg, Sodium 374mg, Total Carbohydrate 35.7g, Dietary Fiber 1.8g, Total Sugars 3.6g, Protein 9.6g

Ingredients:

- 2 cups dry macaroni
- 1 cup of soy milk
- Enough water
- 1/2 teaspoon Dijon mustard
- 1/2 teaspoon salt
- 1/4 teaspoon red chili powder
- 1 cup shredded mozzarella cheese

Procedure:

1. First, add macaroni, soy milk, water, and salt, chili powder, Dijon mustard to the Instant Pot.
2. Now, place the lid on Instant Pot and lock it into place to seal.
3. Pressure Cook on High Pressure for 4 minutes.
4. Use Quick Pressure Release.
5. In the end, stir the cheese into macaroni and then stir in the cheeses until melted and combined.

SPECIAL PLANT-BASED RECIPES

Delicious Jackfruit and Red Pepper Pasta

Servings: 4

Preparation Time: 5 minutes

Per Serving: Calories 110, Total Fat 2.3g, Saturated Fat 0.4g, Cholesterol 0mg, Sodium 168mg, Total Carbohydrate 21.5g, Dietary Fiber 2.5g, Total Sugars 0.6g, Protein 2.3g

Ingredients:

- 1 tablespoon garlic powder
- 1 teaspoon crushed red pepper
- Enough water
- 1/4 cup avocado oil
- 1 cup gnocchi
- 1 bunch fresh mint
- 1 cup jackfruit
- Salt to taste

Procedure:

1. Set Instant Pot to Sauté.
2. Then, add the avocado oil and allow it to sizzle.
3. After, add the garlic powder and cook for 2 minutes. Stir regularly.
4. Now, add jackfruit and cook until about 4 - 5 minutes. Add gnocchi, water, fresh mint, salt, and red pepper into Instant Pot.
5. Lock the lid and make sure the vent is closed.

6. Set Instant Pot to Manual or Pressure Cook on High pressure for 10 minutes.
7. When cooking time ends, release pressure and wait for steam to completely stop before opening the lid.
8. Enjoy.

Servings: 8

Preparation Time: 25 minutes

Ingredients:

- 2 tbsps vanilla extract
- A pinch of salt
- 2 cups shredded coconut
- 1 1/3 cups coconut milk
- 1/2 cup maple syrup
- 4 tbsps cocoa powder

Procedure:

1. Preheat oven to 360 F.
2. Take a pot, place the shredded coconut, cocoa powder, vanilla extract, coconut milk, maple syrup, and salt.
3. Now, cook until a firm dough is formed.
4. Shape balls out of the mixture.
5. Then, arrange the balls on a lined with parchment paper baking sheet.
6. Now, bake for 15 minutes.
7. Allow cooling before serving.

Servings: 12

Preparation Time: 55 minutes

Ingredients:

- 2 tbsps fresh orange juice
- 1 cup plant butter, softened
- 2 tsps ground cinnamon
- 1 cup whole-grain flour
- 1 cup pure maple syrup
- 1 cup old-fashioned oats
- 10 apples, peeled and cut into slices
- 1 cup finely chopped cashew
- 1 1/3 cups pure date sugar

Procedure:

1. Preheat oven to 360 F.
2. Now, place apples in a greased baking pan.
3. Then, stir in maple syrup and orange juice.
4. Sprinkle with ½ tsp of cinnamon.
5. Take a bowl, combine the flour, oats, cashew, sugar, and remaining cinnamon.
6. Now, blend in the butter until the mixture crumbs.
7. In the end, pour over the apples and bake for 45 minutes.

Servings: 8

Preparation Time: 30 minutes

Per Serving: Calories: 263; Fat: 24.1g; Carbs: 9g; Protein: 5.5g

Ingredients:

- 1 teaspoon garlic powder
- 1 cup almond milk
- Sea salt and ground black pepper, to taste
- 6 curry leaves
- 2 (about 100 halves) cups raw walnuts
- 2 slices white bread, crusts removed
- 2 teaspoons onion powder
- 2 teaspoons smoked paprika
- 4 tablespoons olive oil
- 2 tablespoons basil, chopped

Procedure:

1. First, put the almond milk and bread in a bowl and let it soak well.
2. Then, transfer the soaked bread to the bowl of your food processor or high-speed blender; add in the remaining ingredients.

3. Now, process until smooth, uniform, and creamy.
4. Finally, serve with pasta or zucchini noodles. Bon appétit!

Servings: 8

Preparation Time: 10 minutes

Per Serving: Calories: 126; Fat: 9g; Carbs: 8.3g; Protein: 1.5g

Ingredients:

- 3 tablespoons maple syrup
- 10 tablespoons extra-virgin olive oil
- Sea salt and ground black pepper, to taste
- 4 tablespoons chia seeds
- 4 teaspoons Dijon mustard
- 2 tablespoons red wine vinegar

Procedure:

1. First, put all the ingredients into a mixing bowl; whisk to combine and emulsify.
2. Then, let it sit for 15 minutes so the chia can expand. Bon appétit!

Servings: 8

Preparation Time: 35 minutes

Per Serving: Calories: 187; Fat: 13.6g; Carbs: 14g; Protein: 3.6g

Ingredients:

- 8 tablespoons vegan butter
- 4 cups water
- 2 cups oat milk
- 2 teaspoons red pepper flakes, crushed
- 3 pounds turnips, peeled and cut into small pieces
- Kosher salt and freshly ground black pepper
- 4 fresh rosemary sprigs, chopped
- 2 tablespoons fresh parsley, chopped
- 2 teaspoons ginger-garlic paste

Procedure:

1. First, bring the water to a boil; turn the heat to a simmer and cook your turnip for about 30 minutes; drain.
2. Using an immersion blender, puree the turnips with the vegan butter, milk, rosemary, parsley, ginger-garlic paste, salt, black pepper, red pepper flakes, adding the cooking liquid, if necessary.

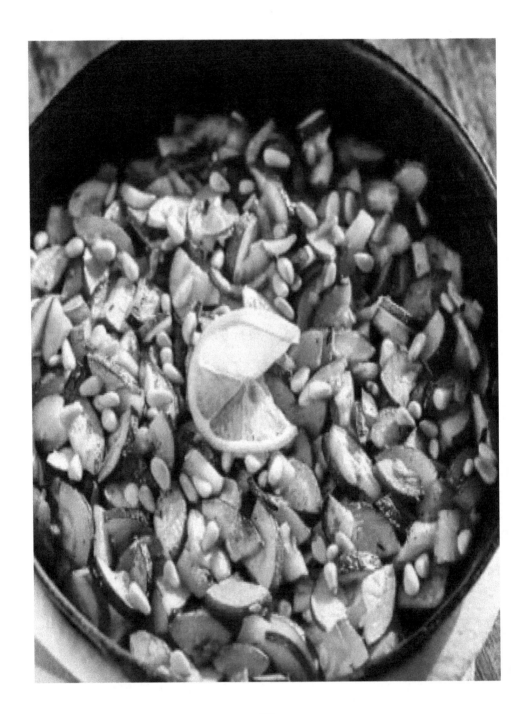

Servings: 8

Preparation Time: 10 minutes

Per Serving: Calories: 99; Fat: 7.4g; Carbs: 6g; Protein: 4.3g

Ingredients:

- 4 tablespoons olive oil
- 4 garlic cloves, minced
- 3 pounds zucchini, sliced
- 2 onions, sliced
- Sea salt and fresh ground black pepper, to taste
- 1 teaspoon dried oregano
- 1 teaspoon dried rosemary
- 2 teaspoons cayenne pepper
- 1 teaspoon dried basil

Procedure:

1. Take a saucepan, heat the olive oil over medium-high heat.
2. Once hot, sauté the onion for about 3 minutes or until tender.
3. Then, sauté the garlic for about 1 minute until aromatic.

4. Now, add in the zucchini, along with the spices, and continue to sauté for 6 minutes more until tender.
5. In the end, taste and adjust the seasonings.

Servings: 8

Preparation Time: 20 minutes

Per Serving: Calories: 338; Fat: 6.9g; Carbs: 68g; Protein: 3.7g

Ingredients:

- 1 cup agave syrup
- A pinch of sea salt
- 1 cup coconut milk
- 4 tablespoons vegan butter, melted
- 2 teaspoons pumpkin pie spice
- 3 pounds sweet potatoes, peeled and diced

Procedure:

1. First, cover the sweet potatoes with an inch or two of cold water.
2. Then, cook the sweet potatoes in gently boiling water for about 20 minutes; drain well.
3. Now, add the sweet potatoes to the bowl of your food processor; add in the vegan butter, agave syrup, pumpkin pie spice, and salt.
4. Continue to puree, gradually adding the milk until everything is well incorporated. Bon appétit!

Easy Tempeh Chops with Caramelized Onions and Brie Cheese

Servings: 8

Preparation Time: 10 minutes

Per Serving: Calories:680, Total Fat:71.8g, Saturated Fat:20.9g, Total Carbs:10g, Dietary Fiber:7g, Sugar:2g, Protein:3g, Sodium:525mg

Ingredients:

- 4 tbsps freshly chopped mint leaves
- 4 tbsps balsamic vinegar
- 2 tsps sugar-free maple syrup
- 4 large red onions, sliced
- 6 tbsps olive oil
- Salt and ground black pepper to taste
- 8 mushroom chops
- 8 slices brie cheese

Procedure:

1. First, heat 1 tablespoon of olive oil in a medium skillet over medium heat until starting to smoke.
2. Reduce the heat to low and sauté the onions until golden brown.
3. Then, pour in the vinegar, maple syrup, and salt.
4. Now, cook with frequent stirring to prevent burning until the onions caramelize, 20 minutes.
5. Then, transfer to a plate and set aside.

6. Heat the remaining olive oil in the same skillet, season the mushroom with salt and black pepper, and cook in the oil until cooked and brown on the outside, 10 to 12 minutes.
7. Now, put a brie slice on each meat and top with the caramelized onions.
8. After that, allow the cheese to melt for 2 to 3 minutes.
9. Carefully spoon the meat with topping onto serving plates and garnish with the mint leaves.
10. Finally, serve immediately with buttered radishes.

Servings: 8

Preparation Time: 10-75 minutes

Per Serving: Calories: 140 Cal Fat: 0.9 g Carbs: 27.1 g Protein: 6.3 g Fiber: 6.2 g

Ingredients:

- 4 tablespoons soy sauce
- 4 tablespoons olive oil
- 1 broccoli head, chopped
- 1 bell pepper, chopped
- Sesame seeds, for garnish
- 1 zucchini, chopped
- 2 handful fresh parsley, chopped
- 1 cup brown rice, uncooked
- 8 garlic cloves, minced
- 2 cups red cabbage, chopped
- 1/4 teaspoon cayenne powder

Procedure:

1. Start by cooking the brown rice as per the package instructions.
2. Bring water to a boil in a frying pan and Then, add veggies and make sure they are fully covered with water.
3. Then, cook for 1-2 minutes on high heat, and then drain the water and set aside.

4. Now, add oil to the wok pan and heat over high heat and Then, add garlic along with parsley and cayenne powder.
5. Then, cook for a minute, stirring frequently and then add the drained veggies, tamari, and the cooked rice.
6. After then, cook for 1-2 minutes and then garnish with sesame seeds if desired.
7. Finally, serve and enjoy!

Homemade Grilled Veggie Skewers

Servings: 8-12

Preparation Time: 10-75 minutes

Per Serving: Calories:680, Total Fat:71.8g, Saturated Fat:20.9g, Total Carbs:10g, Dietary Fiber:7g, Sugar:2g, Protein:3g, Sodium:525mg

Ingredients:

- 4 portobello mushrooms, chopped
- 2 red onions, peeled, chopped
- 2 sweet potatoes, chopped
- Salt and black pepper, to taste
- 4 tablespoons avocado oil
- 8 ears corn
- 4 bell peppers, chopped
- 12 baby red potatoes, quartered

Procedure:

1. First, preheat the oven to 375F and add the sweet potato to a cooking pot along with the quartered potatoes and water.
2. Then, bring to a boil and cook until lightly tender for about 10 minutes.
3. When done, drain the water and let it cool a bit.
4. Now, thread the vegetables onto skewers, and Then, brush them evenly with oil.

5. When done, season the vegetables generously with salt and pepper on each side.
6. Then, cook the vegetables for about 10-15 minutes until tender and cooked through.
7. Afterwards, flip halfway.
8. Now, place the corn directly on the vegetables to cook together.
9. When done, serve and enjoy with the desired sauce.

Servings: 8

Preparation Time: 10-75 minutes

Per Serving: Calories: 140 Cal Fat: 0.9 g Carbs: 27.1 g
Protein: 6.3 g Fiber: 6.2 g

Ingredients:

- 1/2 cup edamame beans, frozen
- 2 limes, 1 sliced, 1 juiced
- 4 spring onions, chopped
- 3 tablespoons vegetable oil
- 2 handful radishes, sliced
- 2 small gingers, grated
- 2 carrots, shredded
- 2 chunky eggplants
- 4 tablespoons soy sauce
- 2 tablespoons caster sugar
- 2 garlic cloves, crushed
- 1 cup jasmine rice
- 4 tablespoons sesame seeds, toasted

Procedure:

1. First, add 2 cups of water to a cooking pan, add rice and salt to taste.
2. Bring to a boil, cook for a minute, and then close the lid.

99

3. Now, reduce the heat to low and cook for 10 minutes until cooked through.
4. Then, turn off the heat and steam for an additional 10 minutes.
5. Now, add a tablespoon of oil to a bowl and toss the eggplant in it.
6. Preheat the wok pan, add the eggplant, and cook for 5 minutes, often stirring until slightly softened and charred.
7. Then, add the carrots to the wok along with garlic, ginger, and spring onions, and then fry for 2-3 minutes.
8. Take a small bowl, whisk the sugar along with soy sauce and a cup of water, and then add it into the wok.
9. Simmer until the eggplant is very soft, for about 10-15 minutes.
10. After, add water to the pan and bring to a boil, and then add the frozen edamame beans, remove the beans, drain and rinse them well under running water.
11. Then, add the radishes to a bowl, drain the beans again, and then add them to the radishes.
12. Now, squeeze lime juice on top and toss well until combined.
13. Lastly, serve the rice in the bowls and then scoop the eggplant and sauce on top along with the beans and radishes.
14. In the end, sprinkle with sesame seeds and garnish with the lime slices. Enjoy

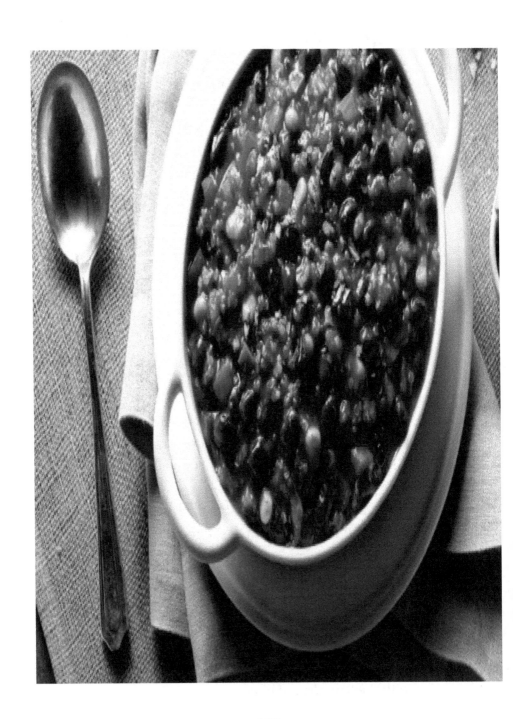

Servings: 16

Preparation Time: 10-75 minutes

Per Serving: Calories: 140 Cal Fat: 0.9 g Carbs: 27.1 g Protein: 6.3 g Fiber: 6.2 g

Ingredients:

- 2 cups quinoa, rinsed, drained
- 2 onions, chopped
- 6 cups vegetable stock
- 2 red chilies, chopped
- 4 teaspoons ground cumin
- 2 lbs of tomatoes, chopped
- Olive oil spray
- 2 teaspoons smoked paprika
- 4 garlic cloves, crushed
- 2 small avocadoes, sliced
- 2 lb. black beans, rinsed, drained
- Coriander leaves, to serve
- 1 teaspoon chili powder

Procedure:

1. Start by generously greasing the cooking pan with oil and place over medium heat, and then add the onion, red chili, and garlic.
2. Then, fry the ingredients until soft, and then add spices and stir.

3. Now, add the vegetable stock into the pan along with quinoa, black beans, and tomatoes, and then adjust the seasonings if needed.
4. Then, close the lid and simmer until quinoa is tender for about 30 minutes.
5. When done, garnish with coriander leaves and top with the avocado slices.
6. Finally, serve and enjoy!

Lightning Source UK Ltd.
Milton Keynes UK
UKHW021822160421
382091UK00005B/57